If you stood alone in the middle of a room covered with mirrors, you would only see yourself. On the other hand, if the room had glass walls, you wouldn't see yourself at all. Instead you would look out at the world.

Every day we make choices—looking inward at our own wants and needs, or looking outward to care about others. Those who constantly look beyond themselves live rich and rewarding lives while they are enriching the lives of others. So if you would like to replace some of the mirrors with clear glass, these four steps may be helpful to you.

AF699741

Four Steps to Abundant CHRISTIAN LIVING

Selma Hudson

A Barbour Book

ISBN 1-55748-987-4

Unless otherwise noted, Scriptures are taken from the King James Version of the Bible.

Published by Barbour & Company, Inc.
P.O. Box 719
Uhrichsville, Ohio 44683
http://www.barbourbooks.com

ecpa Member of the Evangelical Christian Publishers Association

Printed in the United States of America.

Patience

"Love is patient."
1 Corinthians 13:4, NIV

Patience is one of the deepest ways to express love. It paves the way for kindness, forgiveness, and tolerance to take a place in our relationships with others, and becomes a strong force in our lives.

Patience in its purest form is a deep, inner peace, and serenity—a kind of control of thought and action that guards against our being easily ruffled or disturbed. Anger and irritation are the opposite of patience. Proverbs 16:32 says, "He that is slow to anger is better than the mighty; and he that ruleth his spirit than he that taketh a city," and Proverbs 15:18 says, "A wrathful man stirreth up strife: but he that is slow to anger appeaseth strife." Ruling our spirit is what patience is all about, because unruly, uncontrolled thoughts "stir up strife," but calmness and serenity "appeaseth strife."

With patience we can help to dissolve friction and show more love for others, making their lives happier.

Patience comes from within, and we can start with our simple day-to-day experiences. For instance, one day my cat tipped over my knitting bag and started playing with a skein of yarn. By the time I discovered what she was doing, the yarn was in a mass of snarls, some in tiny knots. Unsnarling it seemed a hopeless task, and my first feeling was that I just wanted to throw it out. But that yarn was important to the project I was working on, so I put on a CD of soothing music and sat down with the yarn.

The first thing I had to do was to get rid of any feeling of impatience toward the cat. After all, she did what came naturally to her sense of play, and I had mistakenly left the yarn where she could play with it. So I petted her and assured her everything was okay, though my first reaction had been one of anger. Then I made myself be calm and relaxed, shutting out thoughts about all the other things I could have been doing. Little by little, the snarls and knots disappeared and the ball was whole again. This lesson in patience taught me something very valuable. Because I was calm and understanding, I maintained a loving relationship with my cat (even with animals, irritation can cause hard feelings that make cracks in a relationship), and I realized that patience could make a difference in many situations, not just in dealing with people, but in handling smaller incidents that I could only change by letting God rule my actions and thoughts.

A good place to practice patience is in bumper-to-bumper traffic, when you know you are not going anywhere very soon, or at a traffic light when the light has just turned red. Instead of sitting in your car getting more and more agitated, say a prayer of thanks. Occupying your thoughts and spirit in this way makes time go faster, and does away with imptience. After all, Philippians 4:8 tells us, "whatsoever things are true, whatsoever things are honest, whatsoever things are just, whatsoever things are pure, whatsoever things are lovely, whatsoever things are of good report; if there be any virtue, and if there be any praise, think on these things."

Or try listening to a bird singing, watching a cloud floating lazily across the sky, or closing your eyes for a few seconds and picturing something beautiful. If you think this method sounds corny, just try it and see how much peace it brings to your thoughts and the calm patience you feel. Then you won't be like the impatient people at a traffic signal that make other motorists irritated by constantly honking their horns, cutting in and out of traffic, jumping the yellow lights, or driving through a red light because they don't have the patience to stop. This behavior often causes serious accidents and is sure to make for many angry people.

There are a number of small annoyances that can build into uncontrolled irritation, making it unpleasant for people around you. When waiting in a line, it's helpful to read a book, think about a favorite poem, say something friendly to the person next to you, or be a people watcher. You can brighten someone's day just by having a happy look on your face. Remember, Jesus said, "Ye are the light of the world" (Matthew 5:14). Being a light is a lot better than complaining and making other people miserable.

A friend of mine was waiting in a long line to get her license renewed. She knew it would be tedious and could feel impatience starting to well up in her, so she decided to turn her thoughts to something else. When she noticed the lady behind her looked very unhappy, she smiled sweetly at her. They began to talk and my friend shared some kind words and happy thoughts with her until it was her turn at the window. Then the lady thanked her and told her she felt much better. My friend recalls that the waiting went faster than it ever had before, and she was able to share joy with someone who needed it. My friend found that though impatience breeds irritation and short tempers, when she is patient, it is a blessing to herself and to others.

Another time my friend was in the post office during the holiday season in a long, slow-moving line. There was a man in the middle of the line who was getting more and more agitated. He complained loudly to all those around him, and when he finally got to the window he vented his anger on the clerk, berating her for the poor service. He left with a money order only to come back a minute later, rush up to the window, and yell that the clerk had given him the wrong money order. When the irate man demanded another one, and "NOW!" the clerk patiently told him he'd have to wait his turn. This man was not only rude, he was obnoxious. How much happier everyone in the post office would have been if he had patiently waited his turn.

In our daily contacts we influence the thoughts and actions of others by our patience or impatience. If my friend had grown more and more irritated, making nasty remarks about the inefficiency of government workers and spending her time loudly complaining, the woman behind her could have grown more depressed and felt more negative about her situation. On the other hand, if the man in the post office had patiently waited his turn, perhaps offered to hold packages for weary shoppers (since he wasn't carrying anything), and said an appreciative word to the clerk, at least some people might have left the post office with lighter hearts, feeling the spirit of the season. Since we can never know how we are influencing the feelings of others, it's a good idea to keep watch over our actions, *ruling out* impatience and irritation.

As we develop inner patience in everything we do, we will be more able to express patience toward all those we come in contact with. Cultivating patience will improve any relationship. Being irritable, annoyed, or short tempered sours relationships. Being tactful, sweet, gentle, and willing to listen enriches them. Since we strive to be like Jesus, we ought to be patient with our children, parents, co-workers, spouses, and friends, even if they make the same mistakes over and over. As we are patient and keep our thoughts pure, we will be able to see how we can help others find solutions and overcome their problems.

Impatience can be very costly in our relationships—in the work place, in the home, and in individual self-respect. I know of a factory supervisor who had twenty people working under him. He was very capable and efficient, always got to work on time, worked extra hours without complaining, did things to please his boss, and appeared to be a perfect employee. When an opening came for a department manager he was sure he would get the promotion, but he was shocked when it went to someone else. What happened? Over the years he had worked for the company, the management had received many complaints from his workers about his behavior. He was abrupt and irritable, got upset when they asked questions, criticized individuals in front of other workers, and often left people in tears. Like the parable Jesus told of the unmerciful servant, he did not offer to others the forbearance that he had been granted (see Matthew 18:21-35).

Frank was respected in his community for his volunteer work and other participation in community affairs. Then one evening when he attended a council meeting someone was talking against an issue that he believed in. This person always seemed to be on the opposite side of the fence on the issues that were important to Frank, and he had always managed to keep his impatience and irritation under control. This night, however, something snapped, and he said some very nasty things publicly to his opponent. A dead silence followed, and although no one ever said anything to Frank about the incident, he felt ashamed and lost a part of his self respect.

Carol was a young girl miserable at home. Her parents didn't show her patience at all and complained that she should act more like an adult. When she made mistakes, they got angry and punished her instead of helping her to correct them. When she didn't get high grades on tests, they belittled her. They were constantly irritated and annoyed about things she did or didn't do. Finally she could bear their impatience no longer; when she was fifteen she ran away.

We show the most love for those we care about by patiently letting them grow at their own pace. What's right for them isn't necessarily what we think is right, or at least at the time that we think is right. There is a wonderful example of this in nature, as all of nature teaches patience. As Ecclesiastes 3:1 says, "For everything there is a season, and a time for everything under the sun." Birds build a nest and sit on the eggs until they hatch. Flowers bud and open petal by petal. The process of seed time to harvesting the crops goes in a certain order, and nothing will change it. A farmer prepares the soil, plants the seeds, weeds and cultivates the soil, and when the time is right, harvests the crops. Like the farmer, we prepare the soil of love and patience in which our loved ones grow. It's a precious experience.

Impatience can take a form that keeps others from growing. For instance, because a mother didn't have the patience to teach her daughter to cook, the girl was never even allowed in the kitchen all the time she was growing up. When she grew up and moved away, she literally didn't know how to boil water. She went through many trying meals before she learned to do the most simple cooking. Without realizing it, we can deprive others of valuable experiences through a lack of patience.

In discussing the attributes of love, Paul wrote that love "is not easily provoked" (1 Corinthians 13:5). This is a Christlike characteristic to aspire to—to be undisturbed by the words and actions of others, by circumstances that irritate or annoy, or things we can't do anything about. As Christians we should be patient when a young child asks a hundred questions, to repeat that thing we've already told someone several times, to be patient and kind with slow learners, to be quiet and calm when the impulse is to be loud and angry. A patient Christian can be a soothing balm to uptight, irritated people, and can help bring others a great sense of peace. Some people are like a time bomb, ready to go off at the slightest provocation. What a gift it is to "deactivate" one with patience and kindness!

In its deepest form, patience requires

developing a calm compassion and understanding for the needs of others. In doing this, it's helpful to remember that none of us is perfect, and so others are having to be patient with us. And that, most of all, our heavenly Father is patient with us!

Kindness

"Clothe yourselves with compassion and kindness..."
COLOSSIANS 3:12, NIV

Kindness is more than doing good deeds, it is a deep caring for other people lived out in daily life. It isn't something that is turned on and off, or practiced on special occasions. It is a way of life. Goethe wrote that, "Kindness is the golden chain by which society is bound together." There won't be any chinks in the chain as we constantly live the Golden Rule—treating others as we want to be treated. As Jesus said, "Therefore all things whatsoever ye would that men should do to you, do even so to them: for this is the law and the prophets" (Matthew 7:12).

In Bible times, kindness to strangers was taken for granted, and any deviation from it was almost like breaking a law. A good example of this attitude is shown in the experience of Moses at the well. When seven sisters came to the well where Moses was resting, and after they had drawn water and filled the water troughs, they were chased away by shepherds who wanted the water for themselves. Moses could have stood by and done nothing, but he chose to help the seven sisters water their flock and to protect them from the shepherds. When they told their father about the incident, he asked his daughters, "And where is he? Why is it that ye have left the man? Call him, that he may eat bread." But his kindness begot kindness, and the father showed his gratitude by giving Moses food, a place to live, and one of his daughters for a wife.

This story points to an important truism: that kindness brings its own reward, blessing the giver as well as the receiver. When we give kindness, we always get it back, although not always in ways we might expect.

A young woman named Debbie was persuaded by some friends to spend her vacation at a resort where they expected a lot of single men to be staying. When they arrived at the resort, the friends discovered that the only other guests were older women. Though her friends sulked through the whole vacation,

Debbie befriended several of the older women and spent time doing little things with them, being kind and thoughtful. On the last day of her vacation she was packed and ready to go when one of the ladies knocked on her door. With an unmistakable twinkle in her eye, she said, "Debbie, my grandson came to visit me unexpectedly, and I want you to meet him." A smiling young man took Debbie's hand and said, "I've been hearing a lot about you." It turned out they were from the same city! After several months of dating, Debbie and the young man were married. So you see, simple kindness takes us on many different paths.

Another example of kindness is illustrated in the story Jesus told about the man from Samaria in Luke 10:25-37. Two men passed by a fellow countryman where he lay on the road beaten and stripped of his clothes, and yet they wouldn't be bothered to stop and help him. But a Samaritan who had no relation to the beaten man not only stopped and bandaged the man's wounds, he brought him to an inn where the injured man could be taken care of. But that wasn't all. The Samaritan gave the innkeeper money to care for the man, and promised to give him more when he came back that way. Jesus' parable showed that "neighborly" kindness should be extended in love to all of God's children.

There's another really important thing about being a good neighbor that the parable of the good Samaritan showed. He went all the way, "the extra mile", to make sure *all* the hurt man's needs were taken care of. We must ask ourselves, How good a neighbor am I? Do I "pass by on the other side," too busy or thoughtless to help? Or am I willing to take time to care, even going the extra mile to help others?

One Sunday morning my dad had to go to church early by himself. As he drove along, one of his tires went flat. He got out of the car, obviously dressed for church, and looked with disgust at the tire. Then a car stopped, and a man quickly got out and changed the tire. My dad didn't have much money, but he offered what he had and the man refused. "Sometime do the same for someone else. That'll be payment enough for me," said the man. Then he drove away. My dad never forgot that incident, and has had opportunities to "pay" the man back many times since.

One day I was taking my son to nursery

school when I ran out of gas. I was feeling desperate and alone when a lady stopped and offered to take us to a gas station even though she was on her way to work. When I got the gas, she took us back to our car, and could easily have just dropped us off. But she helped me put in the gas, and made sure I got the car started before she left. This was a great comfort to me.

An exchange student stood on a street corner in New York City looking perplexed. A young man stopped and asked him if he could be of help. The student explained that he was trying to find the subway and was completely confused. Even though the young man was on his way to a class, he said, "Follow me. It might be easier if I show you than if I tell you." He brought the student to the subway where he needed to catch a train, but instead of just leaving him there in the maze of commuter frenzy, he waited until the student got on the right train, before he went on his way. Imagine how cared-for that student must have felt!

These people *lived* the law of kindness, they were willing to pause in their busy lives to help others in need. As these examples show, kindness involves patience, selflessness, and even courage in relating to others. It finds expression in tenderness, gentleness, graciousness, consideration, and goodwill. If these qualities were expressed by all people, the cruel abuses of children, women, older people, and those that are "different" would disappear. Jesus gave us the best example of unselfish kindness. His love of children, patience with his disciples, tenderness with sinners like Mary Magdalene, his provision for his mother's care at the cross, and his compassion toward those with the worst diseases showed a kindness rooted in a deep love. He gave us a map to follow in living our own lives.

As we endeavor to live this kindness, there are many times in the course of our day-to-day lives when we can be good neighbors, and we don't have to do anything dramatic. We can offer our knowledge, experience, or talent. We might take a lonely person to lunch, bake cookies for someone new in the neighborhood who needs a friend, offer to babysit for a tired mother, or help a co-worker who's swamped with work and hesitant to ask for help.

Kindness can be shown in such simple

ways as a kind word, a helping hand, or a warm smile. As Christians we have ample reason to smile, and keep on smiling! Don't be discouraged if people you smile at look grumpy or don't smile back. Maybe they've had a hard day at the office, or had a fight with their spouse, or just heard a piece of bad news. Even perpetual grumps can use a friendly smile to help melt some of the hardness and self-pity in their hearts and brighten their days. Maybe eventually you might even see one smile back!

Sometimes a hug, a gentle touch, or a word of encouragement at the right moment will help a person to know they are loved. Knowing that somebody is willing to listen without criticism or rancor, to understand, and to support can mean so much during a difficult time. Your kindness may give a feeling of worth that can carry someone who is hurting through to better days.

In the simplest form, kindness is a matter of courtesy—it's *listening* to people when they talk instead of interrupting, letting someone into a line of traffic, being quiet when someone is sleeping. It's doing the little things that make others' lives happier.

Kindness ascends the scale of caring into *deeper* thoughtfulness—being supportive instead of ridiculing someone in front of others, being tactful and gentle when correction is needed, doing what someone else wants to do just to please them, looking beyond someone's *words* in regard to how they feel, and sensing their need for comfort. If someone says, "I'm okay, really," do they *mean* it? Sometimes its kind to say, "You know that isn't true. If you don't want to talk about it, that's okay. But if you do, I'd be glad to listen." Letting someone know that you're there for them can be the most comforting thing in the world.

In addition to all the things we can *do* to be kind, another form of kindness that we often don't think of is being careful what we say or don't say about others. A good example to live by is found in the Book of Proverbs, "She openeth her mouth with wisdom; and in her tongue is the law of kindness" (Proverbs 31:26). Keeping guard over one's tongue is one often kindest things one can do. Once something comes out of the mouth, it can't be put back in again. Someone I know learned the rightness of that saying the hard way. My friend was at a piano recital given by several people she knew and afterward was talking to a group of friends about the pianists. She was talking about one of them critically, comparing her to the others, when she discovered the pianist was standing directly in back of her and had heard every negative word she had said. My friend was terribly embarrassed and tried to smooth over the situation as much as possible, but the incident left a very uncomfortable feeling between them. It's always best to find good to speak of others, or else to say nothing. This is following the old saying, "If you can't say anything nice about somebody, don't say anything at all." However, we might ask ourselves, "Are my thoughts as kind as my words?" Acting kind but thinking unkind thoughts is hypocritical and betrays the trust of others. Sometimes we need to decide when its best to be silent or to speak up. Because although it may seem kind to keep silent when someone is being discussed critically, often the kindest thing to do is to add a positive comment to the discussion. Silence may actually add weight to the criticism. On the other hand, gossiping and talking about others behind their back is hurtful and often devastating, and sometimes it's best to keep silent or try to change the subject.

The deepest form of kindness is being kind to unkindness. If someone is unkind or hateful, should we return in like manner? No. Jesus said, "Love your enemies. . . and pray for them which despitefully use you" (Matthew 5:44). When others hurt us, we often feel the im-pulse to retaliate. But retaliation is a form of poison, and never does anyone any good, in-stead it takes away peace and joy. Kindness, however, is never anything but kind, even if it isn't returned. It can dissolve bitterness and hardness. It blesses the giver and receiver (and sometimes even one who observes the kindness) and often changes the life of someone who didn't seem to "deserve" the kindness. It can end up drawing enemies together in peace.

Kindness is felt in the *heart,* not in the *head,* and no one can tell you how to express it. But as you go about living your life, desiring to be kind in your relationships with others, you'll find your own ways to reach out to others.

It can all be summed up with the words of Abraham Lincoln, "After all, the one meaning of life is to be kind."

Forgiveness

"Forgive, and you will be forgiven."
LUKE 6:37, NIV

Perhaps one of the hardest ways to express love to others is to forgive them their mistakes, to even *want* to forgive them their mistakes. But it brings many rewards.

Jesus gave us the supreme example. After spending three years of his life ministering to the needs of others—healing the sick, redeeming sinners, raising the dead to renewed life—he found himself hanging on a cross. What did he do? Did he hate those who nailed him to the cross? No. In a prayer expressing the deepest love he said, "Father, forgive them, for they know not what they do."

Can we say and mean the same prayer when a person wrongs us in some way? And why *should* we? Aren't we entitled to resent or hate those who wrong us? Not if we are living Jesus words, "Love your enemies, do good to them which hate you, bless them that curse you, and pray for them which despitefully use you" (Luke 6:27). Jesus certainly lived what he taught. He never condoned evil—in fact, he gave strong rebuke to the Pharisees and others who hated him. But it's obvious that he never indulged in hate, and didn't seek revenge. This is evident in the passage which tells how one of the disciples cut off the ear of the servant of the high priest. Though the servant was among those who had come to take Jesus away to be tried and killed, Jesus rebuked the disciple who had defended him with the sword and healed the servant's ear. That was a supreme moment of forgiveness toward those who would harm Jesus and a rebuke to revenge.

A story from the Old Testament beautifully illustrates forgiveness. Joseph's eleven brothers were jealous of him because their father loved him best. So first they put him in a pit where he could have been killed by an animal. Then they sold him as a slave. For the next few years he went through some dismal experiences. Among other things, he was falsely accused of attempted rape and put in prison. There he interpreted a dream for the Egyptian Pharaoh's chief cupbearer, who promised to put in a good word for him when he was released from prison, but promptly forgot.

Throughout all the time he had been in Egypt he was betrayed by those that he had done good for. He worked hard, was conscientious and honest. But through the hatefulness or ingratitude of others, he spent years in prison. He didn't hold a grudge or feel resentful toward all those that treated him so badly, or his life would have been a lot different. Because the truth is that resentment or hate unchecked is a poison that affects the way a person thinks and acts, and can eventually destroy the spirit within, leaving an empty shell. Joseph kept growing and becoming a better person because he didn't let the acts of others destroy him.

When at last the chief cupbearer remembered his promise, Joseph was brought out of the dungeon to interpret a dream for the Pharaoh. He interpreted the Pharaoh's dream, and because the Pharaoh recognized Joseph's wisdom and perception, he made him a ruler over the land second only to himself. One day after he achieved this high position, his brothers came to him for help, not knowing that this high ruler was Joseph. The supreme test came when Joseph was face-to-face with them. Because of his position of high power, he could have sent his brothers away without the help they needed. He could have had them arrested. Or he could have even killed them himself. He was in a position to administer swift revenge. What did he do? According to Genesis 45:15, "He kissed all his brethren and wept upon them." And he said, "Be not grieved, nor angry with yourselves, that ye sold me hither" (Genesis 45:5).

This is a truly remarkable story of forgiveness. Not only did Joseph forgive all those who had wronged him in lesser ways, he forgave his brothers who had abandoned him out of jealousy, and also comforted them and didn't want them to suffer for what they did! That is true forgiveness.

Maybe you are thinking, "I can't forgive that way. A person I know did something unforgivable, and I can never forgive him." It may help you to think about what forgiveness is and how it affects our lives. To forgive is "to give up resentment." So forgiveness is putting aside hurt feelings (which often are strongly affected by ego or self pity—"How can he do that to me?" "What will people think?"), hate, and the desire for revenge or retaliation. You can "give up" these feelings by soul-searching to see how you might have done something to prevent the wrong and by realizing that the person who sinned against you may genuinely want to repent and do better. Forgiveness often helps others to recognize their faults and try to correct them, and thereby not repeat their offense.

Forgiveness requires compassion, showing mercy toward the shortcomings and mistakes of others, and being humble enough to know that we all make mistakes. Compassion is looking for the good in others despite any unpleasant qualities. It's being kind in giving someone a second chance. When someone feels another's resentment it often puts them on the defensive and they justify what they did. Mercy melts this away and the person feels shame. This is the first step toward reform, and your forgiveness may encourage that step. Even if your forgiveness doesn't have that effect, your mercy and compassion toward others will bring many blessings.

When you think of the effects of the resentment, giving it up shouldn't be hard to do.

Cherishing resentment hardens the heart and makes us blind to the good around us. A person consumed in their hate and desire for revenge will inevitably end up not showing love to those who love them most. Therefore we owe it to ourselves, our families, and all those who are dear to us to refuse to be hateful, resentful, seek retaliation or revenge, to hold grudges, or rejoice over misfortunes of others. Because forgiveness liberates the forgiver as well as the forgiven.

Forgiveness is not always easy. Sometimes it takes time. It's hard to have compassion for the person who hurt you. But Christians must forgive if they are to become like Christ. Sometimes forgiveness takes place when we recognize the growth that has taken place because of some hurt we have suffered. In enduring pain sometimes we develop qualities—like patience, strength, even faith —that we might not have had otherwise. Remember what Paul said of sufferings: "We glory in tribulations also: knowing that tribulation worketh patience; and patience, experience; and experience, hope" (Romans 5: 3-4).

Susan worked hard to put her husband through college, basically putting her own life on hold. As soon as he graduated, he informed her that he'd been in love with someone else for the ten years they'd been married, and he wanted a divorce. It was a terrible shock to her because Susan thought they had a good marriage. Her husband moved to another state and left her to raise two small children. After the shock and grief wore off, she realized she had a choice. She could become bitter and resentful or she could pick up the loose threads and make a happy life for herself and her children. Instead of resentment, Susan found compassion for her ex-husband. As it turned out, the woman he was going to marry changed her mind. Though he married someone else, for a number of years he struggled with financial problems. His health began to fail, and he seldom saw his daughters, thus missing out on all the joys of watching his children grow up.

Susan, however, went back to college and became a teacher. She had many experiences she wouldn't have had if she stayed married. She had the moral support of friends and family while she went to college and prospered in her new career. Most important to her, she had a beautiful relationship with her daughters that continues to blossom. She never said a negative word about their father to the girls, so they too never felt resentful. The few times when her ex-husband and his wife came to visit the girls, Susan welcomed them into her home as she would old friends, and in time that's what they turned out to be.

Susan's experiences showed her that when someone does something hurtful, they also suffer from their wrong actions. She determined not to ruin her own peace and shut out the good in her life and those she loved by indulging in hate and resentment.

Susan had a lot to forgive. But we can practice forgiveness daily by making the effort to forgive minor hurts, annoyances, and mistakes of others. Such acts of forgiveness may be more important than we realize. Karen was a companion to a very elderly woman who loved classical music. One evening there was going to be a program of opera music on television, and the woman talked all day about how much she was going to enjoy the program. After supper Karen was so busy with various chores that she didn't think to remind her friend of the program until it was over. When she regretfully told her companion that they'd missed the program, the older woman became very upset and berated the young woman for her mistake, and said she'd been denied the one pleasure she had in her "dismal life." Finally Karen said to her, "Marian, why don't you just forget about it and look forward to the next program. It's all past now." Marion answered, "Well, it isn't past for me." Instead of forgiving Karen this oversight, the old lady fostered her resentment, making both herself and Karen miserable. Marion's unwillingness to forgive cost Karen and Marion their friendship. Ironically, though Karen didn't resent the woman's anger, she blamed herself for forgetting to turn the program on. She forgave the woman, but didn't forgive herself. And that is another vital link in the chain of forgiveness.

Another woman cared for her mother after a disabling stroke. This meant lifting the heavy woman without help, being at the beck and call of a bell, and dealing with her mother's idiosyncrasies. It spite of how much the woman loved her mother, so much responsibility was hard on her, and often impatience crept in and sharp words were spoken.

After two years her mother passed on, and the daughter felt an aching sense of remorse. As she began to understand why her mother had said and done some of the things she did, she thought, "Why wasn't I more loving and understanding and patient?" Her resentment toward herself grew until finally one day she said to herself, "I did the best I could under the circumstances. I'm not a trained nurse and I tried to cope. I can't do anything about it, and I'm not going to condemn myself anymore." She was able to forgive herself, and as time went on she had opportunities to help other elderly women in need. If you are mentally kicking yourself black and blue because of some mistake in your past, stop and gently forgive yourself. You deserve to be forgiven as much as anyone else. Jesus forgave you, you should forgive yourself.

If someone you love has said or done something hurtful, it's often helpful to go to that person and explain how it has hurt you. Sometimes people say or do something that they don't realize is hurtful. Or sometimes remarks can often be construed in a way that wasn't meant. Especially if something is told to you secondhand, the best solution is to talk directly to the person who you feel has wronged you. Many hurts can be dissolved through a frank conversation when you give another person an opportunity to present their side of the story.

There are many opportunities in our lives to be unforgiving and many reasons to justify our unforgiveness. But it takes a much bigger person to forgive and truly forget, making individual lives and our world a much better place. A worthy life goal is never to hate or resent anyone, whatever the situation. Instead, "Love one another. As I have loved you, so you must love one another. By this all men will know that you are my disciples, if you love one another" (John 13: 34-35 NIV).

Tolerance

"Be completely humble and gentle; be patient, bearing with one another in love."
EPHESIANS 4:2, NIV

The word "tolerance" sometimes carries a negative connotation, a notion of barely "putting up" with something. And yet the dictionary defines tolerance as "sympathy or indulgence" for something we don't agree with. That makes tolerance a very strong, powerful quality. It goes hand in hand with respect. In the final analysis, tolerance means having respect for each other's differences, whether they might be differences in opinions, looks, abilities, race, beliefs, or culture.

Like compassion, tolerance involves the realization that everyone has something to give, in ways we may not even imagine. When we realize this, we can sometimes take constructive action to help others instead of criticizing them.

There's a great need in the world for a considerate attitude toward the beliefs and feelings of others. We don't have to agree with everybody, but at least we can respect another's viewpoint, listening patiently and respectfully. It's really a kind of humility; rather than insisting on being *right*, or *best*, or thinking the only right way is "my way", tolerance is being willing to really listen and respect others' viewpoints even though we may not agree with them. As Christians, we can disagree without being disagreeable, acknowledging differences and respecting them, being willing to serve instead of rule, and realizing that there's more than one way of looking at things. This humility is very different from rigid willfulness, headstrong obstinacy, or misguided persistence, but is expressed in a quiet acceptance of the different viewpoints of others. This acceptance is not weakness, bur rather a deep inner strength.

In the Sermon on the Mount, Jesus said, "Judge not, and ye shall not be judged" (Luke 6: 37). But we seem to find many ways to judge our fellow beings, sometimes causing antagnism which leads to explosive situations. Exchang-ing judgement with flexibility defuses tense situations and opens the way to compromise—a give and take that can bring a sense of peace and calm that leads to a resolution of differences without a residue of hard feelings.

In conflict situations, often a feeling of superiority can arise, and it may take a big dose of humility to respect the right of others to be different and to respect their need to be respected. This feeling of superiority is illustrated by Jesus' parable about the prayers of the Pharisee and the Publican in Luke 18:9-14. The Pharisee proudly "thanked" God that he was not like other men, but the Publican's wail went out to God for forgiveness of his own sins. The "better than thou" attitude of the Pharisee is the root of all intolerance, so let us all pray with the Publican, and not see ourselves as better than other people.

How often we judge others by our own yardstick! If they do not "measure up" we think they're odd, disgusting, irresponsible, or even dangerous. We make fun of them, or avoid them instead of trying to understand them. The *best* yardstick for our attitudes is to ask ourselves, "How would I want to be treated if I was this person?" So it all boils down once again to the Golden Rule of Matthew 7:12.

Often the judgements we make are irrational, such as that all long-haired people are dirty, lazy, deadbeats; or that overweight people are self-indulgent and undisciplined; or that people of other cultures are strange and not to be trusted. The list could go on and on. Sometimes we pass judgment and don't even try to get acquainted. If we did, we might make some surprising discoveries. Consider what happened in a small, close-knit community. A drifter with long hair and dirty clothes suddenly appeared in the town and spent his time going through the garbage cans looking for returnable cans. The citizens of the town were up in arms and snubbed him completely, never talking to him or showing him any kindness. The man never asked for anything and went about quietly and unobtrusively. At the end of a month he left the town, but not before giving the proceeds of his garbage can rummaging to the three local churches! There were some very ashamed people and a lesson was learned about ways of evaluating people.

We need to realize that when someone doesn't conform to the norm, they are not inferior, nor should they be subject to ridicule. Is a woman from India walking down the street in this country in her sari inferior because she's dressed differently than most women dress in this country? Is someone with a heavy Irish brogue inferior because he talks differently than natives of this country? We should recognize that people of different cultures can enrich our lives as we learn about their traditions and ways of doing things, thus broadening our concepts and our understanding.

When many people recognize differences of any kind in others, they say, "You are not one of us." And, unfortunately, people outside of the norm are sometimes ostracized in the work place, in neighborhoods, clubs, and—worst of all—in churches. Christians can and should set an example of tolerance that can make a real difference in the lives of many.

In the days before desegregation, during World War II, my parents often invited small groups of soldiers from a nearby base to share a modest dinner with our family and spend the afternoon with us. One Saturday they drove past a field after a heavy rain where a number of black soldiers were trying to play football in deep mud. My dad stopped and asked one of the officers if he had ten men who would like to share dinner with them the next day.

"Do I?" he replied with a grin. The next day those soldiers came to our house and brought so much humor and fun with them that everyone had a fantastic time. Through the conversation my mother discovered that two of them went to the same high school she did a number of years before, and even had some of the same teachers. It was a day that was talked about in our home for a long time.

One group in society that people too often look down on and ridicule are those who are overweight. But Christians in particular should make the effort to be understanding and kind. Like Jesus we ought to look past a person's physical appearance and recognize the soul—seeing *the person* within the body for whom Jesus laid down his life.

Recently my friend was sitting alone in a restaurant when a woman came in who weighed at least four hundred pounds. My friend had often felt strong critical feelings for overweight people. But with a new awareness of the Christian attribute of tolerance, she thought, "I don't have a right to judge her. How do I know how much she has suffered?" And so my friend ate her dinner with no more thought of criticism. The overweight woman happened to be seated near my friend, and toward the end of the meal their eyes met and they exchanged a warm, friendly smile. My friend tells me that something special happened in that exchange, and she hoped this woman felt a little less burdened by public opinion. And she knew that she had to change her thought completely about all obese people, in the Christian spirit of love and acceptance rather than the spirit of harsh judgment.

Another group of people who experience a lot of intolerance are the mentally handicapped. Some people seem to feel that because a person is mentally impaired he doesn't have the same needs and feelings as everyone else. When you see someone who is mentally handicapped, remember that his heart and spirit are whole. He still has the same need to be loved, respected, listened to, valued, communicated with, and accepted as you and I. And as we all know, rejection can be devastating.

I was riding a bus one day when a man who was mentally challenged got on. He sat down and said something rather loudly to the man opposite him. I wondered what would happen, fearing the other man might shrink away or brush the young man off. To my relief, the older man answered him, talking and joking with him just like anyone else. I felt a warm glow to see this expression of kindness instead of intolerance.

Our world is getting smaller all the time. With greater international travel and business connections, each of us is experiencing contact with people of differing beliefs, customs, cultures, and traditions. There is a need to understand and respect these differences in order not to offend or anger those of differing backgrounds, or to impose our beliefs on them, to expect them to bend to our beliefs.

An American couple got to know many Japanese people through a sister city program and invited a Japanese couple to visit them. Since the American woman was naturally affectionate, her husband reminded her that since physical contact was uncommon in Japanese culture, their guests would be offended if she hugged them. But through the course of their visits, the four developed a close friendship, and hugging gradually became a part of it. When the American couple went to Japan to visit their friends, the American husband reminded his wife, "Remember, now you'll be in Japan. Don't embarrass our friends by hugging in public, because their friends wouldn't understand and would be offended." When they got to the train station, their friends came to pick them up, and the Japanese gentleman rushed up to his American friends with open arms. They had actually assimilated each other's customs and reached a mutual understanding and expression of caring.

In this diverse world, lives are becoming more and more interdependent, and there is a need for thoughtful cooperation, respecting the unique personalities of all God's children, not feeling better than others for any reason, understanding and listening to others' viewpoints, and acknowledging the fact that everyone has feelings and needs. With tolerance, all of humanity will live together in more peace and harmony.

Patience, kindness, forgiveness, and tolerance. These four steps, learned and practiced, will make us better Christians. Then we might ask ourselves, "Is this a better world because I'm living in it?"

Inspirational Library

[illegible]